CARDIOVASCULAR HEALTH

(UNDERSTANDING FOR PREVENTION OF HYPERTENSION, HEART ATTACK AND STROKE)

BY

AKPOBOME A.

Published by: A&C INNOVATIVE PRINTING PRESS

ISBN: 9798622781605

All enquires directed through whatsapp (+2347052292339)

Dedication

I dedicate this book to the almighty God.

Acknowledgement

I appreciate my parents; Mr. David U. Agadaigho and Mrs. Victoria O. Agadaigho for their pioneer support.

I also appreciate all health students and health workers.

I appreciate most, the almighty God for endowing me with wisdom to write this book.

Preface

This book is written to make all individuals to have understanding of hypertension, stroke, and heart attack, so that they can adequately prevent sudden death and health disaster caused by stroke and heart attack.

Researchers and students that are interested in cardiovascular health will carry out a more intensive research if they chose to start by reading this book.

I have presented seminars on hypertension, stroke and heart attack, but in most cases, it sounds as if I am proclaiming information which will deny individuals from the freedom to eat certain food and will also deny them of the life style they enjoy. I guess it is because they do not have knowledge of what I am presenting.

This book is comprehensive for any individual in any discipline or profession to get at least, a basic understanding for the prevention of hypertension, stroke and heart attack.

Though some terms may be difficult for non-medical practitioners, the **basic understanding** is possible for all and it is very essential for everyone.

I wish you happy reading and healthy life style.

Contents

CHAPTER 1

UNDERSTANDING FOR PREVENTION OF HYPERTENSION

CHAPTER 2

How Gene Mutation Causes Heart Attack and Stroke

CHAPTER 3

UNDERSTANDING FOR PREVENTION OF HEART ATTACK/ HEART DISEASES

CHAPTER 4

UNDERSTANDING FOR PREVENTION OF STROKE

CHAPTER 1

UNDERSTANDING FOR PREVENTION OF HYPERTENSION

What Is Hypertension?

Hypertension is also called high blood pressure; it is a condition that indicates that blood pressure has increased to unhealthy levels.

Narrow arteries and/or increased volume of blood, increases blood pressure to become hypertensive. The narrower your arteries are, the higher your blood pressure will be, this is because the area through which blood is pumped becomes smaller and therefore the blood pressure will increase.

Remember that Pressure = Force/Area

High blood pressure can cause damage to your arteries and other blood vessels.

Understanding the Biology of Hypertension, Stroke and Heart Attack

Blood pressure increases because of two reasons. These are:

1. Blockage and narrowing of blood vessels of the cardiovascular (heart-blood vessels) system.

2. Increase in volume of blood.

If both of the above happens simultaneously, then the blood pressure increases faster and may become as high as to cause hypertension, stroke and heart attack/heart diseases.

Total blockage of the blood vessels carrying blood and nutrient to the heart is called **heart attack,** while total blockage of the blood vessel carrying blood and nutrient to any part of the brain is called **stroke.**

Stroke and **heart attack** result in sudden death or a health disaster that may not be restored to normal till death that is why prevention is better and relevant to all. **Blockage** and **narrowing** of arteries is mainly caused by atherosclerosis. **Atherosclerosis** is the deposition of fats also called lipids (cholesterol and triacylglycerol) on the walls of the arteries. As we proceed, we shall study the genetic influence on the transport and deposition of lipids along blood vessels, by **lipoproteins.**

Increase in volume of blood, and constriction of arteries is caused by stress or a shock, that stimulates the adrenal gland. **Volume of blood** increases faster if the salt (sodium) content of the blood is high. As we proceed, we shall have a better understanding of **genetics in narrowing of blood vessels and increasing of blood volume.**

Hypertension as a Multi factorial Disease

Hypertension is regarded as a multi factorial disease because it is caused by many factors. Factors that may cause hypertension are:

1. Gene

2. Nutrition

3. Environment

4. Activities

5. Disease Condition

6. Shock or stress condition

Types of Hypertension

Hypertension can be classified into two types based on the cause. These are:

1. Primary Hypertension: Primary hypertension is a kind of hypertension that develops over time without any identifiable sudden cause or without a sudden disease condition.

A combination of factors may result to primary hypertension. These are:

i. Gene: Some individuals are genetically predisposed to hypertension. How gene causes hypertension will be explained to you as you proceed. These may be from gene mutation or genetic abnormalities inherited from parents, For example, lipoproteins are genetically produced to transport and deposit (fat) lipids, also secretion of stress hormones and regulation of body fluids and salt (sodium) are genetically stimulated.

ii. Response Of Organ To Physical Changes: Changes in the function of body organs e.g. changes in the function of your kidneys that may lead to increase in blood plasma salt (sodium) and corresponding increase in blood volume due to increase in water of blood plasma, for example change into a stressful condition or change in temperature can also increase blood pressure due to change in function of affected organs.

Please, be vigilant to observe changes so as to make amendments early.

iii. Activity, Nutrition and Life Styles: Your daily activity such as your occupation, your environment, lack of physical exercise and bad nutrition intake that may result to overweight or obesity or high cholesterol food intake, may block your blood vessel, increase your blood volume and cause hypertension.

2. Secondary Hypertension: Secondary hypertension occurs quickly than primary hypertension and may be caused by malfunction of organ(s) caused by a condition. If blood pressure remains high after periods of test and treatment, then your doctor will likely conduct more tests to rule out underlying conditions. These tests include:

i. Urine test

ii. Cholesterol screening

iii. Test of your heart electrical activity

This text will help doctors to detect any secondary cause of your elevated blood pressure, if the condition can be terminated, then the hypertension will disappear.

Causes of secondary hypertension may include the following.

i. Kidney disease

ii. Obstructive sleep apnea

iii. Congenital heart defects

iv. Problems with your thyroid

v. Side effects of medications

vi. Use of illegal drugs

vii. Alcohol abuse or chronic alcohol intake

viii. Adrenal gland problem

ix. Certain endocrine tumors etc.

Genetic Mutation and Biochemistry of Blood Pressure

*Gene expression is the key cause of normal blood pressure, low blood pressure (hypotension), and high blood pressure (hypertension). **Hypotension and hypertension** can cause heart failure, stroke, heart diseases and heart attack. Some people out of a group of individuals in the same environment, taking the same nutrition, having the same activity etc. may become hypertensive and prone to cardiovascular (heart-blood vessels) disease that may result to stroke, heart diseases and heart attack, while others may still have their normal blood pressure.*

Genetic mutation in blood pressure, stroke _and_ **_heart attack_** can be expressed in the following.

1. Transport and deposition of fats (lipids) in the cardiovascular system.

2. Adrenal Glands

3. Brain

4. Kidney

The expression of gene in any of the four above will affect the blood vessels' space through which blood flows, the volume of blood; amount of fat deposited on the blood vessels, increase in blood volume, and constriction of blood vessels are all coordinated by the gene.

1 Transport and Deposition of Fats in Cardiovascular System:

Gene synthesizes molecules known as lipoproteins (LP) and it is responsible for the transport of fats along blood vessel, the lipoprotein is the combination of a protein and a fat total.

The three lipoproteins are:

i. High density lipoprotein (HDL)

ii. Very low density lipoprotein (VLDL)

iii. Low density lipoprotein (LDL)

i. **High Density Lipoproteins (HDL):** *High density lipoprotein (HDL) is thought of as good cholesterol because it lowers ones risk of atherosclerosis. HDL is involved with phospholipids metabolism and it has high percentage of protein. HDL is responsible for the removal of cholesterol from tissues and therefore has high capacity to dissolve a great percentage of cholesterol. HDL is anti-atherosclerosis and therefore prevents coronary heart disease.* **Coronary heart disease is** *a condition that is caused by fats accumulation that blocks the blood vessel that carries blood to the heart; this is as a result of deposition of fats due to high level of low density lipoproteins (LDL) in blood of some Individuals.*

Individuals with high level of HDL will not experience atherosclerosis or coronary heart disease, because the HDL transports lipids for metabolism and not for deposition into blood vessels. HDL enhances the utilization of cholesterol in the body for the synthesis of steroid hormone, pile and pile acid salt, which enhances the digestion of fats (lipids).

ii. Very Low Density Lipoprotein (VLDL): VLDL is the medium for transport and deposition of endogenous lipids, especially the triacylglycerol.

iii. Low Density Lipoprotein (LDL): LDL is the medium for the transportation of cholesterol along blood vessels and it is pro atherosclerosis and therefore promotes coronary heart disease, **LDL** is referred to as bad cholesterol.

Individuals with gene that elevates LDL and VLDL are associated with increased risks of atherosclerosis and cardiovascular diseases.

2. Adrenal: Adrenal gland secretes **adrenalin** and **aldosterone** which is secreted by adrenal cortex. **Adrenalin** prepares the body for emergency condition or stress. Individuals with over secretion of this hormone (adrenalin) will become more hypertensive than individuals that have normal secretion even if both experience the same stress condition.

During stress, **adrenalin** increases heart beat so as to increase blood and nutrient supply to produce energy for an emergency condition. The volume of blood is increased, blood vessels constrict, and blood pressure is increased during stress. Adrenal cortex hormone; Aldosterone is a chemical (hormone) that regulates the amount of salt in the body; it is a very specific compound responsible for maintaining the concentration of sodium and potassium inside and outside the cell. This in turn has a direct effect on the amount of fluids in the body and the blood pressure.

Aldosterone is manufactured in the adrenal cortex under direction of another hormone called ACTH (adrenocorticotrophic hormone). ACTH is produced by the anterior pituitary gland, and it stimulates the adrenal cortex to secrete a wide variety of hormone including aldosterone as well as cortisol.

As the concentration of aldosterone rises in the body, the concentration of sodium and water rises, thus more fluid is retained in the body and blood pressure rises during stress or shock condition. **Individuals that secrete high level of aldosterone will therefore have high blood pressure. On the other hand individuals that secrete low aldosterone have lower blood pressure in the same stress condition.**

3. Brain: *The anterior pituitary gland of the brain secretes a hormone (adrenocorticotrophic hormone which controls the renin-angiotensin-aldosterone system (RAAS), as mentioned earlier, aldosterone is part of the RAAS that is responsible for regulating and maintaining sodium balance in the body. Dietary sodium restriction stimulates RAAS activity, while sodium loading reduces the RAAS activity.*

The brain therefore has regulatory systems to maintain appropriate levels of blood pressure, cardiac filling volume, blood volume and potassium/sodium balance in the body. **Mutation in gene or inheritance can cause impairment in function of these hormones in individuals, may increase or reduce blood pressure in individuals.**

4. Kidney: *The kidneys are responsible for the long term regulation of blood pressure through a system of chemical substance or hormone called the rennin-angiotensin-aldosterone system (RAAS), in response to either potassium or angiotensin. The steroid aldosterone is released from the adrenal glands. This hormone is able to rebalance the potassium excretion, sodium and water retention, and regulate blood pressure. For those suffering from* **adrenal fatigue,** *as the adrenal continues to* deteriorate, aldosterone which is the hormone responsible for regulation of amount of water and blood flow in the body, also diminishes. **As sodium and water flow decrease as a result of reduced aldosterone in the body, blood flow, drastically slows, also lowering your blood pressure. On the other hand, as renin-angiotensin-aldosterone is over secreted in some individuals, their blood pressure also increases.**

Kidney function is therefore responsible for high blood pressure, low blood pressure, as well as normal blood pressure in various human.

Adrenal Fatigue and Low Blood Pressure

Adrenal fatigue is a condition that is largely caused by stress and it is a process where the adrenal is exhausted because of stress and is unable to mount a compensatory response. Typical blood pressure of a person in adrenal fatigue ranges from normal blood pressure and high blood pressure in early stages and then progresses to low blood pressure in later stages. In this case the blood pressure usually drops below normal as the compensatory mechanism fails. Aldosterone is a hormone secreted by the adrenal cortex, which is part of the rennin-angiotensin-aldosterone system (RAAS), which regulates blood *pressure. Cortisol is a hormone that is secreted by the adrenal cortex under the direction of Hypothalamus-Pituitary-Adrenal (HPA) axis and is a main anti-stress hormone. Low aldosterone and cortisol levels may cause **adrenal fatigue** and the **adrenal fatigue** also lowers the aldosterone and cortisol which leads to a more low blood pressure symptoms. When the blood pressure drops, blood flow to the brain reduces and the person becomes dizzy and lightheaded. **Adrenal Fatigue** causes dehydration due to respond to high blood pressure in its early stage; this is over body response to over constriction of blood vessels. Taking more fluid can be quite helpful in the majority of essential hypertension cases in its early stage. Later stage of adrenal fatigue is reduced blood pressure when blood vessel relaxes and the adrenals are exhausted.*

How to Understand Blood Pressure Readings

Two numbers create a blood pressure reading.

These are:

1. Systolic blood Pressure: This is the first number and it indicates the pressure in your arteries when your heart beats and pumps out blood.

2. Diastolic Blood Pressure: This is the second number and it is the reading of the pressure in your arteries between beats of your heart.

Categories of Blood Pressure Reading

1. Healthy Blood Pressure: A healthy blood pressure reading is 120/80mmHg (millimeters of mercury).The above blood pressure reading indicates that, the systolic blood pressure is 120mmHg and the diastolic number is 80mmHg.

2. Pre hypertension: This is when blood pressure is between 120/80mmHg and 139/89mmHg. At this stage the doctor advices you to adopt a healthy life style to help lower your blood pressure. As you proceed you will understand such healthy life styles.

3. Stage 1 Hypertension: This is when blood pressure is between 140/90mmHg and 159/99mmHg.

4. Stage 2 Hypertension: This is when blood pressure is above 160/100mmHg. This is very dangerous and is a sign of an advanced stage of hypertension. Further diagnosis is required to detect any secondary cause or a complicated primary cause of hypertension.

Treatment of High Blood Pressure (Hypertension)

The type of hypertension you have determines the treatment option for your hypertension based on the cause.

Primary Hypertension Treatment Option:

Primary hypertension can be treated with a healthy lifestyle that suits your gene and environment. Your doctor should recommend drugs and counsel you regularly

Secondary Hypertension Treatment Options:

Doctors will recommend drugs to treat the cause of secondary hypertension and hypertension treatment drugs. For example, a hypertension caused by kidney disease will be treated by both hypertension relief medications + medication to cure the kidney malfunction. Some medications to cure a particular disease may also increase the blood pressure of some individuals; the doctor prevents such hypertension by trying alternative drugs that will not increase blood pressure. Cases like pregnancy can also increase blood pressure.

Blood Pressure during Pregnancy

Women with hypertension can deliver healthy babies despite having hypertension.

Some women may develop hypertension during their pregnancies; this condition is called **gestational hypertension,** it often reverses itself once the baby is born. Some pregnant women also experience low blood pressure.

Symptoms of High Blood Pressure

High blood pressure is a largely symptomless (silent killer) disease condition. You can only discover that you are hypertensive, if you check your blood pressure regularly. If you ignore your blood pressure because you think a certain symptom or sign will alert you, then you are taking a dangerous risk.

However, people with high blood pressure will experience symptoms like, **nervousness, sweating, difficulties in sleeping, dizziness, blood spot in eyes, facial flushing, headaches, or nose bleeds** etc., but all these symptoms are also symptoms of other disease conditions.

In conclusion, regular blood pressure testing is the true and sure way to detect hypertension in all individuals.

Low Blood Pressure (Hypotension)

Blood pressure tends to be lower if blood volume is too low or if less blood is being pumped into the arteries, also abnormal dilation of arterioles also slow flow of blood.

If blood pressure is too low, it may damage vital organs such as brain, brain cells, and heart because of insufficient blood flow to supply oxygen and nutrients to these organs and the person may feel lightheaded, dizzy and even faint.

Prevention of low blood pressure is by increasing the volume of blood and prevention of **adrenal fatigue.** Individuals with adrenal fatigue experience a more complicated and prolonged **low blood pressure**

Prevention of High Blood Pressure (Hypertension)

Prevention is possible through **home remedies** and **dietary recommendations**.

A. Home Remedies for High Blood Pressure: Healthy lifestyle can help you to prevent hypertension. Prevention is far better than cure, because it is easier to reverse **hypertension** than **stroke** or **heart attack**. The most common home remedy includes:

1. Developing a healthy diet: A healthy diet is vital for helping to reduce high blood pressure. It is also important for managing hypertension even with medications, reducing the risk of complications of hypertension prevents stroke, heart disease, and heart attack.

A heart-healthy diet emphasizes food that includes:

i. Fruits

ii. Vegetables

iii. Whole grains

iv. Lean protein like fish

v. Avoid food that contain no egg yolk, red meat and over fried oil; don't fry oil during cooking if you are prone to hypertension, but if you must fry, just use onion to make a very slight frying.

Dietary recommendations for people with high blood pressure: One of the easiest ways you can use to treat hypertension and prevent possible complications is through your diets. What you eat can go a long way in easing or eliminating hypertension. The most common dietary recommendations for people with hypertension include:

a. Eat less meat but more plants: A plant-based diet is an easy way to reduce the amount of sodium and trans-configured saturated fats you take in from dairy foods and fried meat. Increase the amount of fruits, vegetables, leafy greens, and grains you are eating. Substitute the amount of red meat for healthier lean proteins like fish and poultry.

Note: If you are above 50 years, I advise you not to eat food like **red meat**, and **eggs** because they contain high level of cholesterol that may be deposited on the walls of your blood vessels, which may generate into **atherosclerosis** and may result to **hypertension**, **stroke** and **heart attack.**

Remember **atherosclerosis** is a condition caused by accumulated lipids (cholesterol + triacylglycerol) deposited in blood vessel walls which forms plague that narrows the blood vessels.

b. Reduce dietary sodium: People with high blood pressure and those with an increased risk for heart disease should aim to keep reduce or avoid salt. The best way to reduce sodium intake is by avoiding processed or prepackaged food which are also high in sodium.

c. Avoid sweet food: Sugary foods and beverages contain empty calories but do not have nutritional content, if you want something sweet, try eating fresh fruit, honey or small amount of chocolate that contain no sugar. **Studies suggest eating dark chocolate reduces blood pressure.**

2. Increasing physical activity: Reaching a healthy weight should include been more physically active. In addition to helping you reduce weight, exercise can help reduce stress and lowers blood pressure naturally, and strengthen your cardiovascular system.

Aim to exercise at least 150 minutes of moderate physical activity each week, that is, about 30 minutes daily for five times per week.

Exercise and adequate rest is a great way to manage stress.

3. Reaching a healthy weight: If you are overweight or obese, losing weight can help to lower your blood pressure.

4. Adopting a cleaner lifestyle: If you are a smoker, try to quit, tobacco damages and hardens blood vessel walls by increasing **atherosclerotic blood clotting.**

If you regularly consume too much alcohol or you are used to drinking alcohol, seek help to stop drinking alcohol.

Both smoking and alcohol increase oxidative stress and consequently complicating atherosclerosis to form clots that may even block the blood vessels and may result to stroke and heart attack.

Other activities can also be helpful. These include:

i. Medication

ii. Deep breathing

iii. Massaging

iv. Muscle relaxation

v. Getting adequate sleep

Medications for High Blood Pressure

Note: Always consult your doctor before taking any medications on hypertension; it is dangerous to take blood pressure pharmaceutical drug medication without a physician. All of the pharmaceutical drugs medications used to treat hypertension should be prescribed by a medical practitioner after a blood pressure check.

CHAPTER 2

HOW GENE MUTATION CAUSES STROKE AND HEART ATTACK

The genetic cause of stroke and heart attack is mainly attributed to the high level of blood low density lipoproteins (LDL) that deposit excess cholesterol in the blood which accumulates in blood vessels and leads to blockage of blood vessels. The main cause of heart attack and stroke is **hypercholesterolemia** (high blood cholesterol), which is the genesis of atherosclerosis. The other genetic cause is the adrenal gland that can over secrets stress hormones that causes abnormal increase in the volume of blood and the corresponding over constriction of blood vessels, all these lead to hypertension.

Hypercholesterolemia (high blood cholesterol) can be caused by the rate of synthesis of LDL, rate of degradation of LDL, and rate of removal of LDL from the blood.

Individuals with familial hypercholesterolemia have mutations in the gene for LDL receptors that bind and transport cholesterol to the lever for degradation. Individuals with heterozygous genotype for the mutation have fewer functional receptors and thus remove less circulating LDL particles than a normal *individual. Individuals with homozygous genotype for the mutation have no receptors and thus cannot remove circulating LDL particles.*

There is another genetic observation that has to do with a certain gene called PCSK9. Mutation in PCSK9 is another inherited form of hyper cholesterol in blood. PCSK9 is a soluble protein involved in degradation of LDL receptor. Individual with homozygous genotype for PCSK9 are free from the mutation.

Strategies for Reduction of Hypercholesterolemia

1 Avoid Cholesterol Diet: When we eat less or no cholesterol diet by saying no to egg yolks, red meat, and milk etc., LDL in the blood will be reduced.

2 Avoid Saturated and Trans Fat: Saturated lipids are found in bad oil that can easily become solid at room temperature, they are also found in margarine (butter), over fried oil produces trans-configured fat and we can easily and mistakenly consume them from fried food. This strategy 2 will work together with strategy 1 above.

3 Use Bile and Binding Resin to Draw out Cholesterol: This is one of the medical processes to reduce LDL in the blood.

4 Statin Drug (HMG-COA Reductase Inhibitors): This drug will reduce LDL in the blood drastically.

Why We Need Little or No Cholesterol Diet As We Grow Older

Cholesterol consists of about 50% of the cell membrane and it is the precursor for the synthesis of sterols hormones including the male and female sexual hormones. Every growing child and adolescent needs reasonable quantity of cholesterol in their diets for growth and synthesis of sexual hormones for optimal development of their reproductive system and general body development. As we become older: we stop to grow, so the synthesis of cell membrane stops, our reproductive system is no more developing and we need little or no sexual hormone because aging reduces sexual activity. Consumption of cholesterol at old age is useless and dangerous as it will lead to hypercholesterolemia which eventually leads to atherosclerosis because it will result to **hypertension, heart attack and stroke.** Only people that have a gene that is favorable to degrade and excrete excess cholesterol as explained above will escape the danger of excess cholesterol consumption. Please always check your blood pressure to discover if you have any genetic mutation that can cause hypercholesterolemia and stop imitating people's nutrition because you may not escape the danger linked to the kind of gene you have.

CHAPTER 3

UNDERSTANDING FOR PREVENTION OF HEART ATTACK AND HEART DISEASES

What Is Heart Attack?

A **heart attack** is a health condition that occurs when there is a complete blockage of an artery called coronary artery that supplies oxygenated blood to that area of the heart.

Heart attack is mainly caused by a ruptured atherosclerotic plaque which forms clots that completely blocks the blood vessel, remember atherosclerosis in in chapter 1.

As you get older, the smooth inner walls of the arteries that supply the blood to the heart can become damaged and narrow, due to the buildup of fatty materials called plaques and are formed from atherosclerosis. When an area of plague is ruptured, blood cells and other part of the blood stick to the damaged area and forms blood clots that cause blockage of blood vessels. **Food from fried oil and alcohol etc., that induces oxidation, has been proved to be responsible for this rupture of atherosclerotic plaque.**

A heart attack occurs when a blood clot completely blocks the flow of blood and seriously reduces blood flow to the heart muscles. This also results in patient's previously experiencing chest pain called **angina** before occurrence of heart attacks.

Causes of Heart Attack

Heart attack can be caused by many factors which include all the causes of hypertension. Please go back to chapter one for the causes of hypertension. **Research have shown that the main cause of heart attack and stroke is from gene mutation coupled with bad nutrition such as; taking diet rich in cholesterol, consuming food produced from over fried oil, drinking alcohol or** engaging in smoking; are high risk factor of heart attack and stroke, because they increase oxidative stress which result in conversion of atherosclerotic plaque to clots, that blocks the blood vessel.

Coronary Heart Disease (CHD); A Stage before Heart Attack

Coronary heart disease *is a common cause of heart attack. It has been that before any case of heart attack, there has been existing coronary heart disease that has existed in weeks, months or years.*

Atherosclerosis *is the pioneer cause of heart attack by narrowing and blockage of blood vessels.* **Coronary Heart Disease (CHD)** *is caused by cholesterol and fat deposition been deposited in the walls of the arteries that supplies nutrient and oxygen to the heart, these deposits, leads to narrowing or constriction of the blood vessel, thereby resulting in hypertension. From the laws of physics, pressure is the outcome of force per given area (P=F/A) so that the heart exerts more pumping force or given pressure (since pressure is directly proportional to force) so as to supply itself with oxygen and nutrients. Before this condition is experienced, the heart is said* _to be experiencing high blood pressure. Like any organ, the heart needs a constant supply of oxygen and nutrients, which are carried by the coronary arteries. Fixed narrowing that is often calcified (hardened) usually cause angina (chest pain). Less severe narrowing may contain unstable blockages called atherosclerotic or fatty plaque and the condition is known as atherosclerosis. Unstable atherosclerotic plague can rupture, resulting in clot formation, no blood flow, and a heart attack occurs._

It would be stressed here that if enough oxygen carrying blood is blocked from reaching the heart, you may experience a type of chest pain called **angina.** However, if the blood supply to a portion of the heart is totally blocked off by total blockage of a coronary artery, the result is **heart attack.** This is usually due to a sudden closure of the artery by a blood clot forming on top of unstable plaque.

Symptoms of Heart Attack

Some symptoms of heart attack are:

1. Chest pain

2. Lightheadedness

3. Nausea

4. Extreme fatigue

5. Fainting

6. Dizziness

7. Pressure in upper back

8. Discomfort in your arm(s), shoulder(s) neck, jaw or back.

9. Feel short of breath

Prevention of Heart Attack

1 Please go back to chapter one for prevention of hypertension, prevention of hypertension is the first step to prevent heart attack.

2. Always be vigilant to discover any of the above symptoms of heart attack and take fast action by consulting your doctor.

3. Check your blood pressure regularly and ensure it is kept normal at about 120/80mmHg always.

CHAPTER 4

UNDERSTANDING FOR PREVENTION OF STROKE

What Is Stroke?

Stroke may also be called brain attack especially if it is caused by total blockage of the blood vessel that supplies blood and nutrients to any part of the brain.

Stroke is a health condition in which the cells of any part of the brain lacks blood and nutrients, whereby causing the brain cells to die and the corresponding paralysis of that part of the body been controlled by that part of the brain with dead cells.

Types of Stroke

We have two types of stroke. They are:

1. Ischemic Stroke: This is the cause of most strokes. Ischemic stroke is a stroke that is caused by total blockage of the blood vessels that supplies blood and nutrients to any part of the brain. This is also called **brain attack.**

Mini Stroke: A transient ischemic attack or TIA is also known as a mini stroke, except that the symptoms last for a short amount of time and no longer than 24 hours. This is because the blockage that stops the blood from getting to your brain is temporary. A temporary decrease of blood supply to any part of your brain causes TIAs, which often last less than five minutes.

2. Hemorrhagic Stroke: This is a stroke caused by bleeding in or around the brain. This kind of stroke is not common and is caused by break in the wall of a blood vessel. This causes blood to leak into the brain, again stopping the delivery of oxygen and nutrients.

Hemorrhagic stroke can be caused by a number of disorders which affects the blood vessels, including long standing high blood pressure and cerebral **aneurysm.** An **aneurysm** is a weak spot on blood vessels; the weak spots that cause aneurysms are usually present at birth.

Aneurysm develops over a number of years and usually do not cause detectable problem until they break.

Causes of Stroke

Heart attack and **stroke** happen after hypertension is complicated to the extent of total blockage of important blood vessel(s) in the heart or brain respectively. The most effective cause of stroke is through atherosclerosis and also increase in volume of blood caused by excess salt (sodium) and stress, this starts with hypertension and eventually stroke if not prevented. Once stroke has happened, the damaged is almost always irreversible except a condition caused by mini stroke. A stroke occurs when the blood supply to your brain is interrupted or reduced. This deprives your brain of oxygen and nutrient, which can cause your brain cells to die.

A stroke may be caused by a blocked artery **(ischemic stroke)** or the leaking or bursting of a blood vessel **(hemorrhagic stroke).** Some people may experience only a temporary disruption of blood flow to the brain **[transient ischemic attack (TIA) or mini stroke].**

Causes of Ischemic Stroke

About 85% of strokes are ischemic strokes. **Ischemic stroke** occurs when the arteries to your brain become narrowed or blocked, causing severely reduced blood flow (ischemia). The most common ischemic strokes include:

1. Thrombotic Ischemic Stroke: A thrombotic ischemic stroke occurs when a blood clot forms in one of the arteries that supplies blood to your brain. A clot may be caused by fatty deposits (plaque) that build up in arteries and cause reduced blood flow (atherosclerosis) or other artery conditions.

2. Embolic Ischemic Stroke: An embolic ischemic stroke occurs when a blood clot or other debris forms away from your brain. In most cases, the blockage is in your heart and is swept through your blood stream to lodge in narrower brain arteries. This type of blood clot is called an embolus.

Causes of Hemorrhagic Stroke

Hemorrhagic stroke occurs when a blood vessel in your brain leaks or ruptures. Brain hemorrhages can result from many conditions that affect your blood vessel including uncontrolled high blood pressure (hypertension), over treatment with anticoagulants and weak spots in your blood vessel walls (aneurysms). A less common cause of hemorrhage stroke is the rupture of an abnormal spot of thin-wall blood vessels present at birth.

Types of Hemorrhagic Stroke:

1. Intra-cerebral hemorrhage: In an intra-cerebral hemorrhage, a blood vessel in the brain burst and spills into the surrounding brain tissue, damaging brain cells. Brain cells beyond the leak are deprived of blood and also damaged.

High blood pressure, trauma vascular malformations, use of blood-thinning medications and other conditions may cause an intra-cerebral hemorrhage.

2. Subarachnoid Hemorrhage: In a subarachnoid hemorrhage, an artery on or near the surface of your brain bursts and spills into the space between the surface of your brain and your skull. This bleeding is often signaled by a sudden severe headache.

A **subarachnoid hemorrhage** is commonly caused by the bursting of a small sack-shaped or berry-shaped outpunching on an artery known as an aneurysm. After the hemorrhage, the blood vessels in your brain may widen and narrow erratically *(vasospasm), causing brain cell damage by further limiting blood flow.*

Risk Factor of Stroke

A. Lifestyle and Nutritional Risk Factor of Stroke:

i. Been overweight or obese

ii. Physical inactivity

iii. Heavy or binge drinking

iv. Drinking alcohol, smoking or use of illicit drugs such as cocaine and methamphetamines

v. High Cholesterol consumption

Medical Risk Factors of Stroke:

1. **High Blood Pressure:** If your blood pressure is above 140/90 mmHg, it is said to be high. Keep it normal at about 120/80mmHg.

2. **Cardiovascular disease:** These include heart failure, heart defects, heart infection or abnormal heart rhythm.

3. **Diabetes:** Diabetes induces oxidative stress which causes the atherosclerotic plague to rupture and forms blood clots that blocks the blood vessel carrying blood to any part of the brain.

4. **Obstructive sleep apnea:** This is a sleep disorder in which the oxygen level drops during the night hereby preventing sound sleep.

Symptoms of Stroke

1. Trouble with speaking and understanding.

2. Paralysis or numbness (weakness) of the face, arms or legs.

3. Trouble with seeing in one or both eyes

4. Headache

5. Trouble with walking: You may stumble or experience sudden dizziness, loss of balance or loss of coordination.

Prevention of Stroke

1. Please go back to chapter one for prevention of hypertension. Prevention of hypertension is the pioneer step for prevention of stroke and heart diseases.

2. Avoid the above risk factors so as to prevent hypertension, stroke, heart attack and other cardiovascular diseases.

3. Always be very vigilant to discover any of the symptoms of stroke and take fast action by consulting your doctor.

4. Check your blood pressure regularly and ensure it is kept normal at about 120/80mm

REFERENCES

Kimberly Holland (2017). Health Line (Everything You Need TO know About High Blood Pressure (Hypertension).

Dr Lam (2016). Body. Mind. Nutrition (Signs And Symptoms: Low Blood Pressure Causes And The Correlation With Adrenal Fatigue.

Dr Lam (2016) Body. Mind. Nutrition (Adrenal Fatique And Blood Pressure Symptoms-Part 1).

Melissa Conrad Stoppler MD. (2017). MedicineNet.com (12 Heart Attack Symptoms and Early Warning).

Nwaka A.C And Uzoegwu P.N (2008). Bio-Research, 6(1): 323-327

Yoko W, Momoko Y, and Hiromichi Y (2015). International Journal Of Molecular Medicine